The Health Literacy Guide to Aging with Style:

Tackling those tough aging questions with grace!

Introduction

Welcome to my first book based on Health Literacy and Health Living. I decided to write this series, which are all based on classes I teach in New York and Massachusetts, to bring this crucial information into the country. The first three chapters of this book will explain a lot more about Public Health (I am a public health educator), Health Literacy, and Health in general. As more of these books are written, you will notice that these first three chapters do not really change. That is because it does not matter in what order you pick up the books, you still need this background information to understand why these are not your ordinary healthy living books.

These books are designed to start conversations—between you and your family, between you and your medical team, between you and your employer. They will provide more questions than answers because everyone has different health needs and therefore different answers will be the right set of responses for you and your family. And the answers will change over time because your health changes over time.

In the age of the internet, I will not share all my history and how I got to be here in this introduction. If you would like to know more about me as a professional, you are welcome to check out my LinkedIn page where I am listed as Karen Burhans Laing.

I also want to take a moment and thank a few people who helped me get here. Donna Smith and Carrin Swanson were early believers in my classes for seniors and Donna especially challenged me to create many new classes for her memory care center. Alyssa Plock was invaluable at getting my book up and printed. And a big thanks to Chris Milian of Albany NY Premier Aerial Photography for the apple tree photo on the front and back cover of the book.

In the meantime, I hope this book gets you thinking and talking. If you have questions, you are welcome to email me at info@healthliteracyforall.org, but the answers to your questions will mostly come from you. This is the essence of health literacy, your ability to make good every day decisions about your life based on your health and your experiences.

Be Healthy!

Karen Laing

Chapter 1: What is Public Health?

"Good Afternoon, My name is Karen Laing and I am a public health educator. Does anyone know what public health is?" I use this opening line in every class I teach. Unless I am teaching in a community that hires me regularly, I am usually met by blank stares and a lot of head shaking. And why would you know what public health is? It is the hidden side of the medical system. The prevention piece of the US Healthcare system which works well for some, not at all for a few, and okay for most. Public health studies death, dying, and illnesses to help Americans to live as long as possible with minimum disability.

From the public health side of medicine, there are five areas of sub-specialties. The first is the research division, also known as epidemiology. These researchers are often found in state and federal health departments and they are the people who put out the contradictory test results, like coffee is good for you, coffee is bad for you, coffee is good for you. At this moment, research shows the drink one makes from coffee beans is good for you...as long as you don't smoke cigarettes with it, dunk donuts into it, or put tons of cream and sugar into it, and if your body can handle the caffeine that naturally occurs within the coffee bean.

The coffee research is a great example of why research is often contradictory and further studies often need to be done. Public health does not want to assume anything; it needs to prove that the core issue and not anything else is responsible for the results. So when coffee was first deemed bad for you, there hadn't been a close look at the research taking out the effects having a cigarette with your coffee. Cigarettes have been proven over and over again to be horrible little sticks of destruction, and once the results separated out the coffee-only addicts vs the coffee-and-cigarette addict, coffee seemed healthier. When studies separated out those who drank coffee but paired it with highly un-nutritious food (like donuts and desserts), coffee again improved in the health realm. And again there was a difference between those who drank their coffee black, those who only used a little flavoring, and those who liked "a little coffee with their cream and sugar." Then finally, research got to an individual level. How did *your* body process the caffeine? If you can't handle caffeine, then coffee might be just fine for your neighbor and no good for you. Just like strawberries are great, unless you are allergic to them, then you should not eat them.

Once the statisticians in the research field are pretty sure they can link a cause and effect together, they will often send the research to the second division- public policy. This is where that research goes to creating laws to keep us safe. Fluoride in drinking water, and seat belt laws are two of the US's most well-known public health policies or laws.

The environmental health section, the third division, made a huge impact in the clean air and water acts from the 60s and 70s as well as more recently with fracking and Legionnaire's disease prevention. While I was editing this book, Hurricane Harvey hit Houston. Houston is a city known for very few grassy areas (green space as it is called in public health.) Environmental health was already aware that the more green space there is, the healthier residents and employees tended to be. Perhaps because nature has a calming effect on people, perhaps because there is extra oxygen in the atmosphere from the plants. Now, with no green space in Houston, there is nowhere for the water to go to. Estimates are it could be as long as two months before the water recedes/evaporates. I am sure the environmental public health division will be closely studying the effects on the buildings and people's health when the water floods a building and city for two months in comparison to the areas around Houston that had the same intensive rain, but had green space for the water to be absorbed into the ground. Look for public policy to start changing laws about the amount of green space needed for building in a year or so (the end of 2018.)

Biotechnology is the fourth subdivision. Current technology is studied and continuously improved upon. Oxygen tanks that were highly combustible, heavy, and very limiting to how far a senior could go with it have been replaced with oxygen concentrators that are lighter weight, have little risk of exploding and simply need to be plugged in to work. The lighter weight equipment combined with the increased safety has seriously improved the daily lives of those who need extra oxygen to live. Again, one can see the public health focus toward allowing people to live as full a life as possible despite the chronic illness they live with.

Finally, I come to the last specialty area—social, behavioral and community health. How does public health change a large society to live healthier lives? One of the ways public health does this is through vaccine clinics in stores that make it convenient for people to be vaccinated. Or through public health educators who run trainings to help people understand their illnesses better. Since I started this book with the comment, I am a public health educator; you can see that this is my specialty. I train, less on specific diseases, but on a set of core values called "Health Literacy."

Chapter 2: What is Health Literacy?

According to the US government health literacy is "the degree to which individuals have the capacity to obtain, process, and understand basic health information and services needed to make appropriate health decisions." In other words, it is a core set of skills YOU need to navigate the healthcare system (in sickness and in health), make healthy decisions at home, and (I have included) respond in a public health emergency. Health Literacy is understanding the ABCs of the healthcare system. Most public health educators teach on specific diseases, I teach on skills and knowledge that underlie those diseases.

Health literacy, like financial literacy, is a concept we are just beginning to recognize as key to a successful long life. If you don't know the basics of balancing a checkbook, you are inevitably going to bounce some checks along the way. If you don't understand the how and whys of taking medications (for example), you will make mistakes and end up potentially harming yourself or others.

In the United States, it is estimated that only 1 out of 10 Americans is proficient in health literacy skills. And when the mental health system is involved, the numbers go down to 1 out of 33 patients. The US medical system first recognized that patients were not fully health literate in the 1980s. Back then AIDS patients and Breast Cancer Patients both began demanding the right to be involved in their own care. They wanted to make decisions about treatment and lifestyle choices and when to end treatment. As doctors handed patients over the right to make decisions, they realized that not all patients could make the right decisions. Medical schools taught doctors to use "plain language," translators, and to provide education guides with pictures. While this was a good step toward better communication, it did not solve a patient's ability to ask questions and feel competent to make decisions. It changed the doctor's way of communicating, but did not improve the health literacy skills of the patients.

In 2012, I found myself studying health literacy for a college internship. I was asked to design a tool to help a poverty-based agency screen which of its clients needed training in health literacy. It did not take long to realize that since only 1 in 10 people were health literate, the answer was not to screen, but to train everyone. I then researched what was available to train on health literacy skills. Since it was 20 plus years since the US had identified the problem, I thought it would be easy to put together some trainings for the everyday patient to use. Sadly, that was not the case. The public health sector was still fighting over whether health literacy included skills or knowledge, as well as how to assess patients' abilities to navigate. As a retail trainer for years and a special education teacher to start my career, it made more sense to me to start training people and see how that improved health literacy skills. And so I created the first health literacy training program in the country designed to teach everyone on these basic skills. I used the bits of curriculum I could find from cancer, heart disease, and diabetes education, along with my training as a researcher to read through the latest research. I wanted to find the pieces of knowledge and define the communication aspects that would help patients clearly share with their doctors about their health concerns, needs, and values.

When I started my work, only California taught directly to patients, and they taught only to low income parents who used Medicaid. By the time I was done with my internship, Florida had also developed a program under its English as a Second Language program. A year later, Minnesota began teaching to seniors. To the best of my knowledge, we are the only four programs focused on teaching skills directly to patients anywhere in the world even now 5 years after I started researching this. The rest of the country and the world is still trying to correct a patient deficit by retraining medical providers. In 2016, the agency I helped open won an Award from the New York State Public Health Association for Outstanding Leadership in Public Health for our work as Health Literacy advocates and trainers.

So why is it crucial that people have good health literacy skills? According to the federal report Inadequate Health

Literacy A Barrier to Patient Care, patients who do not have good skills struggle unnecessarily and at a high cost. They are

1. More likely to report poor health status
2. Twice as likely to be hospitalized
3. Remain in the hospital more days per each admission
4. Have 1 more outpatient visit per year
5. Have more difficulty using metered inhalers
6. Have worse HbA1c levels (blood sugar levels)
7. More likely to make medication errors
8. Less likely to comply with recommended treatments.

As a result, they are more likely to be seriously disabled or die at an earlier age than someone with excellent health literacy skills. According to the National Action Plan to Improve Health Literacy, lack of health literacy skills costs the United State between $106 and $236 billion annually in medical bills alone, and an additional $238 billion in wasted medications. As you can see, it is important that public health get to the hard work of teaching Americans to improve their health literacy skills to help control medical expenses as we simultaneously help people live longer.

Chapter 3: What is Health?

Within the first few minutes of every presentation, I like to ask the questions, "What do you think health is?" and "Are you healthy?" Most people answer the first question with comments like, being able to do what you want, getting out of bed in a good mood, exercise, eating fruits and vegetables. In other words we tend to think of health as a primarily physical thing with a bit of a mental health piece to it. But according to the World Health Organization, health consists of physical, mental, social and spiritual health. It is important that we look closely at all four aspects of health.

Most people have a pretty good idea of what physical health encompasses. Physical health is why one would see a medical doctor. It includes illnesses and disabilities. Each of us are born with a certain health level and for the rest of our lives, we make decisions to, hopefully help us stay that healthy or even get healthier. Exercise, enough sleep, good nutrition, avoiding bad habits, and learning to reduce stress are all included in the decisions made at home that reflect in the medical tests for issues like cholesterol, cancer, blood pressure and blood sugar levels. As seniors, It can becomes harder and harder for them to think of themselves as physically healthy when their physical bodies naturally can do fewer and fewer things.

Most people have a fairly straight forward understanding of mental health, too. Right now, advocates are in a national push to change the term from mental health to behavioral health. Behavioral health includes minor problems like anxiety and grief and a general outlook on life, up to more serious issues like learning disabilities, drug and alcohol addictions, schizophrenia, and Alzheimer's disease. At any time one's mental health can take a serious dive. For some people it can return to normal with a little bit of help, or can lock a person in a world of confusion that is hard to escape. One in four will have a problem with their mental health at some point in their lives, but not all of the problems are long term, chronic diseases. As seniors age, their mental health tends to stabilize unless they develop some form of age-related dementia.

Social health is the aspect of health that as Americans, we often think about the least. It includes how we get along with others, as well as how others get along with us. The ability to hold a job, save for the future, make friends, raise a family, and enjoy the world are all aspects of social health. When physical health wanes in our old age, what keeps seniors happy and optimistic is their social health. Seeing their family and friends, living in a community with other seniors who are also socially healthy, having enough when they retire to make their lives easier, all offset the physical limitations of struggling to walk or hear or see as well.

Spiritual health is an area that we, as Americans, often do not discuss at all for fear of insulting others. Spiritual health is where one finds their inner strength to get through the bad moments of life. It is their personal beliefs that help them reach the end of their life feeling that they lead a purposeful life. It forms a core set of values on which people make decisions, including health choices.

Spiritual health and physical health decisions should work together to help people be at peace about what they are doing. No one should put their personal values to the side when making medical decisions. This is one of the crucial areas where health literacy training comes into place. If someone does not want to take a medication or get a blood transfusion because it violates their spiritual values, they need to be able to share that with their doctor in such a way, that the doctor looks for alternative ways to treat that patient. It's not about ignoring the disease or being non-compliant. It's about balancing all aspects of your health. The same is true of social health. Many seniors will continue treatments past the point they are comfortable with, simply to keep family members happy.

When health literacy skills and all four aspects of health are taught to seniors, they can have the end of the life they want to live. As long as they are willing to open up and explain to their doctors, families, and others, how their values and their treatments intersect to either bring them peace or restlessness. Ultimately, everyone wants to live at peace with others and with themselves. And this is why one cannot ignore one's physical health, but one must balance it with their mental, social and spiritual health: and then be able to share that information comfortably.

Chapter 4: What is Aging?

I like to look at aging as a process that builds to a climax and then slowly goes away. Babies start out with almost no skills whatsoever. They use their ability to scream and cry to get the care they need. Soon though they learn social skills to get what they need: they laugh, point, and stare to make their needs known. In the first two years of their lives, they learn to talk and walk, develop social cues and connect with their parents to create stable mental health. As children reach their fifth year of life, they know almost everything they need to survive. One of my favorite books was called *All I Really Need to Know I Learned in Kindergarten* by Robert Fulghum. His list of key life skills are:

1. Share everything.
2. Play fair.
3. Do not hit people.
4. Put things back where you found them.
5. Clean up your own mess.
6. Don't take things that aren't yours.
7. Say you're SORRY when you HURT somebody.
8. Wash your hands before you eat.
9. Flush.
10. Warm cookies and cold milk are good for you.
11. Live a balanced life - learn some and drink some and draw some and paint some and sing and dance and play and work everyday some.
12. Take a nap every afternoon.

13. When you go out into the world, watch out for traffic, hold hands, and stick together.
14. Be aware of wonder. Remember the little seed in the Styrofoam cup: The roots go down and the plant goes up and nobody really knows how or why, but we are all like that.
15. Goldfish and hamster and white mice and even the little seed in the Styrofoam cup - they all die. So do we.
16. And then remember the Dick-and-Jane books and the first word you learned - the biggest word of all - LOOK."

This list outlines keys tips to growing up healthy and well and it works until about 50. Then things start to become harder to do. Most people after 50 have experienced the death of at least one close family member, and have developed at least one chronic disease. As one gets to the last fifteen years of their lives, they often struggle with physical health. Hearing and vision loss isolates them from the rest of the family. The health choices they made when they were younger have impacted their bodies and they now struggle with 2 or more chronic illnesses. They may not walk as stably, taste food the same way and may not breathe as well as they did when they were younger. In the last two years, our hearts and bodies slow down at a more intensive pace. Everything seems to go at once. The problem with aging is that while one can clearly define the first two and five years, it is virtually impossible to identify the last fifteen years and the last two years until one is at the very end of their live. Then family can often look back and say, "He was totally fine until *this* happened and then it was all downhill from there." Often that spot is something that happened just about two years earlier.

Ideally this book will help you and your family to make decisions that will improve your own last few years or the last few years of your aging family member. By openly discussing these difficult aging questions early and often, everyone will be involved in decisions based on the senior's health concerns, not just their physical ones, but their mental, social and spiritual ones as well. In 2001, the Center for Medicare and Medicaid looked at the last year of life finances. It showed that the US spent 17% of all Medicare expenses in the last year of someone's life. This is because doctors are using more costly treatments and more surgical and hospital time in the last year of life than any other time in the post 65 aging process. Why is that important? Because most people don't want to spend the end of their lives in and out of hospitals and nursing homes. They do not want to die in a cold sterile hospital bed away from family, but Medicare expenses show that is exactly how most people end up dying. Perhaps this is because, as Astro-Zeneca Chairman David Brennan said once, "Americans have a funny approach to this -- we think death is optional." Sadly, it's not. Just like aging is not. So we might as well do our best to understand the process so we can live out our lives in the last two years, the same way we did the first 80. Balancing all aspects of health and having a good time doing so!!!

Chapter 5: Help is NOT a Four-letter Word

We have all seen it. That moment when we knew we couldn't help someone in time. The car accident that has come out of nowhere. The child falling off her bike. These moments often replay in our brains as we struggle to adjust our lives to the fact that we cannot fix everything. Or perhaps you can help someone but they will not let you. The toddler trying to put on his own shoes. Your neighbor, a victim of domestic violence, who denies that she is being abused—despite the fact that you can see the black eye and you heard the fight.

We are Americans. We were raised to be independent, but also to be willing to help others. Parents taught us to share, hold doors, and be respectful of our elders. We could not survive growing up without mentors and friends to light the way. We thrive on the concept that it takes a village to raise a child. We expect when we give advice to the next generation they will take it as a golden nugget – they may or may not- but we expect it anyway. As we get older, we talk more about the importance of politics or religion and other topics that young people don't discuss because they fear offending others. And we don't care anymore, we know these topics need to be talked about.

Then we turn 65. Or 75.

And we forget that we need to guide our family through this portion of life's journey. We hide how much pain we are in, that we are not able to care for ourselves the same way, that we fell twice last week and it scared us.

We also forget we can ask for help. Help to change light bulbs, mow the grass, and clean the windows. Slowly, things that took us no time at all when we were young, take us all day; and then take us two by the time we recover. We start refusing invitations to outings because it's too noisy and we cannot hear well. We stop going out at night because we don't see well at night. But we don't say that. We say no. We don't give people the chance to help us. We may even begin to bounce checks or leave the stove on. Things that could be truly detrimental to our lifestyle or our safety, but we are too prideful to share with our family members. Senior Americans think it's ok to live alone and isolated because they are independent. But that may not be the best thing for them, in fact it seldom is.

The sad thing is from the perspective of the 50-year-old, we aren't stupid. We can see our parents age in front of us. We have noticed that the once spotless yard is now a bit of a mess. We can tell you don't walk as well and we may even notice the bruises from falling. But you are our parents. You have guided us, taught us to tell the truth, and now you are hiding things from us. And we may be afraid of starting the conversations. "You need some extra help," becomes a phrase we do not want to say at all. Help becomes a four-letter-word on both sides of the discussion. Unlike when we are younger and refused help and it was simply frustrating, seniors put their lives at risk when they refuse the help.

So what are those issues that come up in every senior's life? Things that they will need help with eventually. Things that are easier to talk about before we reach the point where the senior refuses all help. A study in Life Science shows that when children spend too much time in isolation from others, their brain changes and becomes unable to learn and process. When a senior lives in isolation, there is a similar effect that also contributes to fear of the outside world, including allowing "outsiders" into their house to clean or for them to move to a new location where isolation is less a factor.

In New York we have two basic system issues that make our seniors in more danger. One is that we have laws that protect our senior's rights to make their own decisions right up to their untimely death from a bad decision. Our adult protective services do not remove seniors from unsafe situations. Children need to get their elderly parents declared incompetent if they want to help a parent who won't take their medications or who sign up for every Nigerian prince's offer to send them a million dollars. It's hard to prove incompetence and who really wants that fight with their parent.

Secondly, because we have these laws, hospitals are required to treat everyone over the age of 18 the same. In other words, if they would send a 45-year-old patient home from the ER at 4 am with a diagnosis of bronchitis and an antibiotic, they will also send the 95 year old home at 4 am with the same script. HIPAA prevents hospitals from calling family members to discuss whether the 95-year-old is safe at home. She came in alone. She says she is safe. So she is. So home she goes, alone, at 4am, with a script and bronchitis. With potentially no way to leave the house tomorrow to get the medication. These are issues that public health is starting to look at and find better solutions to, but right now, they make it harder to provide good care to a senior who has decided that any help is a four-letter-word.

We are going to use the rest of this book to explore some of these issues. Like any other system of care, some of the advice found in here will apply to New Yorkers only, but it won't take long for a non-New Yorker to find out what the system is like in their state. Check with your county or state Office for the Aging. Ask about the questions we bring up here with senior specialists in your area. In the meantime, you can begin the discussion with your family about what is best for both the aging senior in your family and the family itself.

Chapter 6: Common Senior Frauds

Home Improvement Scams

Most everyone is aware of the home improvement scams that seem to target the elderly every spring and summer. Contractors will come by and say the roof needs repair, offer to repave the driveway, or will legitimately bid on a home repair project and take the money and not do the work. These same scams are tried on younger people, but we are not home as often to fall for them, or we have the energy to take the scammers to court or press charges for criminal court. These are the nightmare stories that scare seniors from letting reputable businesses into their homes and lives.

When my kids were growing up, I pretty much had a policy if my kids wanted to go somewhere with friends, I was going to say yes. With four kids, I appreciated when they were given an opportunity to do something that we might not be able to afford or that appealed to enough of us to do. As a result, my kids needed a way to express themselves so I would say, "No." when they didn't want to go. Ultimately, as a parent they needed me to be the bad guy sometimes. They didn't necessarily want to have to say to their friend, "I don't want to." Or maybe they had and the friend pushed the issue. So we decided that when they did not want to do something, they phrased the question a little different. Instead of saying "Mom, can I go?" they reworded it to, "Mom, I can NOT go to this event, can I?" That was my cue to say "No, you cannot go." No matter how much they begged, or their friends begged, I knew to protect my kids' true feelings by continuing to say no.

Now I suggest that seniors use their kids as a similar shield for the world. When approached by someone looking to pave your driveway or repair your deck, etc. simply say, "I like to humor my kids and let them 'approve' all my spending choices. If you would leave the info here, I will share it with them when they visit and then I will call you." Scam artists will walk away without leaving any paperwork. They will tell you that they are only in the neighborhood at that moment, so they can give you a good deal. But they will not wait around for approval from your kids. The same "trick" works on telemarketers. Legitimate ones will mail you paperwork for your kids to look over, scammers will hang up.

Telemarketers, Contests, and Internet Scammers

Again, because seniors are more likely to be home (or not to use their cell phones to screen their calls), they are also more likely to be the victim of these scammers. Contests like, "Send us $100 and we will process your winnings!" still impact seniors every year, at a higher rate than younger people. And even the internet scams like email from the IRS demanding back taxes will rattle the most stalwart senior into doing something foolish. Requests from overseas charities or fake charities are all too common. For every one that gets through to a younger person, there are two or three that make it to the average senior. I cannot tell you how many times I got an email from a local bank, asking for me to call or respond by email to them because my account is now "inactive," "frozen," or "in jeopardy of being closed." Except I never had an account with that bank. I ignore those emails. But seniors, especially women whose husbands used to do all the banking before they died, are susceptible to those frauds. Are they sure their husband didn't have an account? So they call or respond and give their social security number without thinking about it.

Again seniors should use their children as shields. Showing them the letters, emails, and information gathered on the phone call, helps to protect the senior from making a rash decision. Scammers are good at making it sound like the world will end if you do not respond now. Seniors, with a desire to "handle the problem themselves," often fall into the trap. Ideally, seniors should have a child or grandchild on their accounts, helping them to ensure they are managing everything ok. Setting this process up while the senior is still highly competent to make their own decisions is ideal. Then as they age they will tend to use the system of showing you everything first and they will be less likely to make a really bad financial move on their own.

The Grandparent Scam

This is one of the nastiest scams, and grandparents that fall for it are often re-targeted again and again.

A young adult will call a senior and start the call with "Hi Grandma. It's your favorite grandchild! How are you?" Within a few moments they are telling "their grandma" this horrible story about the car breaking down, or that they were arrested while on vacation. Then they ask grandma to wire them money to get the car fixed or to bail them out of jail. Sometimes, they can take Grandma's check or credit card over the phone, but these scammers are much more likely to have grandma go to Wal-Mart and complete a Western Union wire transfer. It is so common that Wal-Mart now trains their associates to ask questions about where and why seniors are sending money across the country.

Often this scam works best on seniors whose families are dysfunctional. The grandchild often begs grandma not to say anything to mom and dad. They may have a sob story about being abandoned by the boyfriend that the parents didn't like. Or that they got in a fight with the parents just before they left on vacation. Or even that mom and dad, "just hate me and won't do anything for me." Grandma may be so interested in having a relationship with a grandchild she hasn't seen in a while and will send the money hoping the child will come visit. The more isolated the grandparent is from the family; the more likely this scam is to work. And to work over and over again until the fake "granddaughter" has drained all the funds from the grandmother's account.

In all three of the above scenarios, the scams work best when the senior is isolated and alone most of the time. A socially active healthy senior is more likely not to fall for these schemes, either because the family is helping him/her avoid them or because they are talking to friends who can alert them to when fraud is going on in their area. Making sure your senior loved one doesn't fall for any of these scams is key to keeping them safe- financially, but also mentally.

Identity Theft

Identity theft occurs with seniors just the same way it does with others. As anyone who has ever had their identity stolen knows there is often nothing you could have done to prevent it, nor anything you did to cause it.

However, there are two unique problems that come with identity theft in the elderly. First seniors don't use their credit like younger people do and they tend to have great credit. They are not likely to buy a new car or even open a new credit card: things that might alert a younger person that they were the victim of identity theft. It is crucial that someone is checking the senior's credit report as regularly as one does as a younger person.

The second problem that comes with identity theft for seniors is when they pass away. If a senior dies with debt from identity theft still outstanding, that debt will need to be paid from their estate like any legitimate debt. Since they cannot testify that they did not create the debt, it is considered legal debt. So far, this statute has held up, even when the senior lived in a nursing home or memory care center during the creation of the debt; even when the debt was created in another state or country. Laws may eventually catch up with reality, and you need to check if you do not live in NY to see if this is true in your state. In the meantime, this problem goes away if someone is just consistent with checking the credit score and correcting any mistakes on it.

Chapter 7: Understanding Your Doctor's Orders

Understanding a doctor's orders includes many more health literacy skills than this book will cover. This topic can (and probably will) be its own book someday. In order to keep this to a quick guide, I am going to provide just a couple of basic tools to help.

Bring a Date to the Doctor

Seniors over 65 should always bring someone with them to the doctor's office with them. Medical information can change in a single appointment and it can become complicated quickly. Most people over 65 have at least one medical concern and often have two or more. The person who goes with the senior should be in the doctor's appointment with the patient and feel comfortable enough to ask questions. Whether the senior chooses their spouse, their best friend, or one of their children, there needs to be a level of comfort between the senior, the date, and the doctor that allows all three to have an open conversation and ensure that everyone agrees on what the patient will be doing at home to keep themselves healthy.

While there may be a time a senior ends up at a doctor's office without their companion, no one over 65 should ever leave a hospital alone. Really, no one at all should leave an Emergency Room alone. So often, the hospital is where one enters in distress, waits to be seen until the distress has either nearly killed them or the wait itself has. After all the tests, one is sent home with a new diagnosis or treatment and the exhaustion and pain levels often stop one from getting all the discharge information down. As I said earlier, hospitals are obliged to treat all patients the same way, so it is the senior patient who must call their doctor date when they go to the hospital and ask for that person to join them. And they must refuse to be discharged until their friend is there to make sure that everything is safe.

It's Not Safe

As a little extra trick, in New York State, hospitals are not allowed to send a patient home to an unsafe environment. So if someone is being discharged and there is the potential for a problem, the phrase one wants to use "I do not think she will be safe in her home if you release her now." The key word in that is SAFE. Once that word is out there, the hospital is required to have a social worker ensure the patient is safe to go home. Whether that means arranging for home care, making sure the patient has someone who can get the new medications, or just that there is someone from the family at the house who can help the senior get in and settled.

Keep Notes

Ideally, everyone should have a medical notebook that allows them to keep notes. Nowadays, many doctor's offices have online patient portals that will allow the patient to see their latest test results, their prescriptions, and any other details of their medical treatments. There is often a space where patients can email a question or upload additional information. But if a patient has multiple doctors, or a complicated medication or treatment regiment, it is often helpful to keep notes that go from one doctor's office to the next.

New York created a program called HIXNYS. HIXNYS is an online tracking system that links most doctor's offices, urgent care centers, hospitals, and pharmacies medical records. As more organizations join the system, it allows one medical office to review a patient's records from another office. I am a huge believer in using HIXNYS, as one's latest medical records are immediately available to all medical providers. This makes keeping up with a single patient's medical records, labs, medications and treatments easier for providers. One can sign up in your primary care doctor's office.

Use the Teach Back Method

The "teach back method" was originally created by the medical system to make sure the patient understood the doctor. It takes about three to four minutes to do and the patient literally "teaches back" to the doctor or nurse everything he learned during the appointment. The patient can do this or the "doctor date" can. It gives the doctor a chance to correct any information that the patient has wrong or for the doctor to further explain something the patient may be confused about

To use the method, the patient waits until the end of the appointment then says, "When I get home, my loved one/daughter/noisy neighbor will ask what happened at the doctor's office today. If I tell them this ________________ (fill in the blank with what you think happened in the office), will I have missed any crucial information? Your doctor should be able to tell you, "yes you have that all right," "you have most of it right, but this part," or "no, let's go over it all again." If the doctor has to reteach the patient and doctor date anything, they should re-teach the doctor again until his answer is "yes, you have this all right."

This is a great time for you to make sure your notes are up to date and make sure that any corrections the doctor makes to your knowledge is written in your note book. You will want your doctor date to make notes on anything you missed or had wrong.

The teach back method is outlined in the graphic on the next page.

Teach Back Method

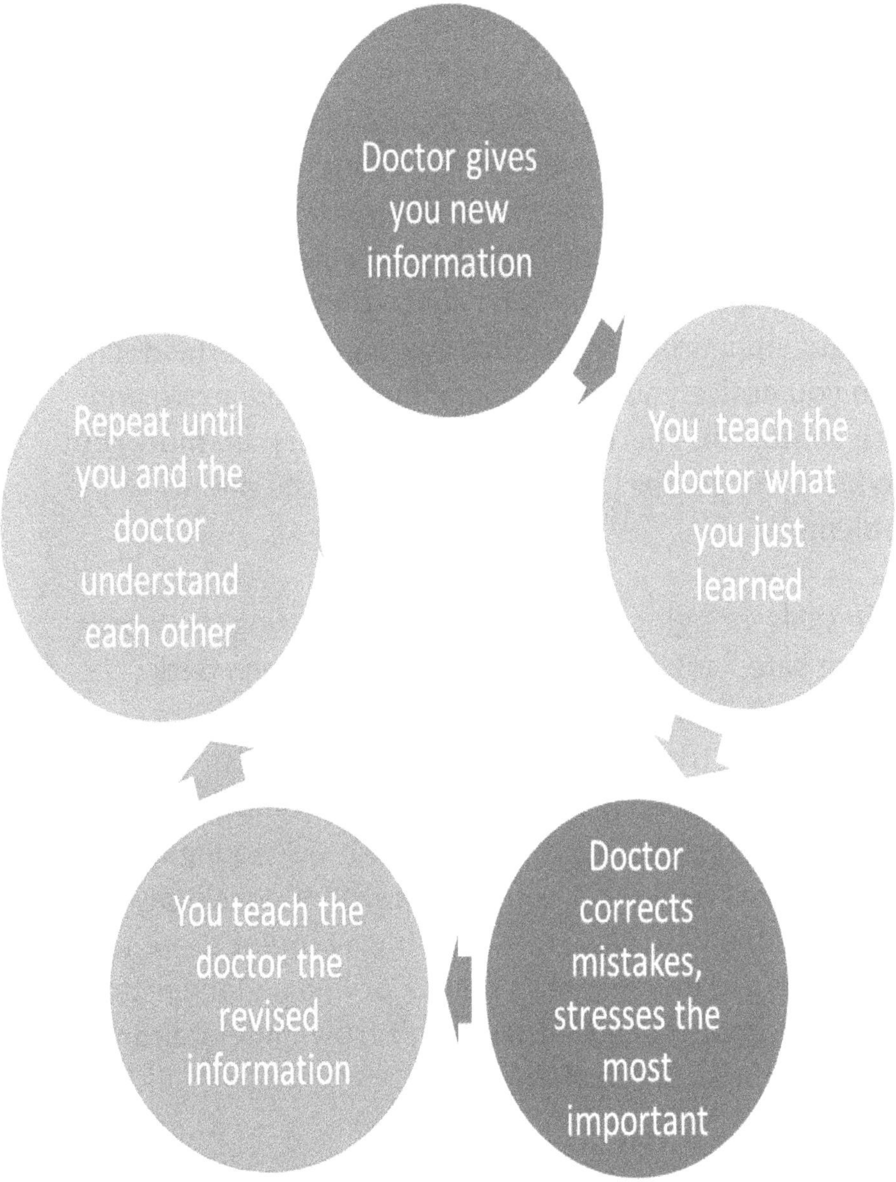

If you are the senior's doctor date, you should be paying attention to how often the patient has the info wrong. Hopefully, you start as the doctor date when the senior gets it all right. Over time though, it will be inevitable that the patient will miss more and more information. Perhaps this is because he is dehydrated, losing health literacy skills from the number of illnesses he's navigating, or there is a bit of dementia appearing. Make sure you mention to the doctor when you notice your senior beginning to have more and more confusion. This is when you should step up more, but also have the doctor look for a reason for the memory problems.

These skills, bringing a date to the doctor, using the words "it's not safe," taking notes, and using the teach back method, are all crucial for seniors to be sure they are understanding their doctor well. They should also be used by younger people managing two or more chronic illnesses, or one life threatening illness. Parents with sick young children may also want to bring a non-parent with them simply to have someone with less emotional involvement there to hear the doctor. INo one wants to be sick or in pain longer than necessary simply because they didn't truly understand what their doctor was telling them.

Chapter 8 Managing Medications

One of the biggest issues in health care is the use of medications. So I want to start this chapter by playing a game called what is the medication?

Question 1: You struggle with anxiety. The doctor wants to give you a prescribed anti-anxiety pill that you can only buy at the pharmacy. The massage therapist say, "Try St john's Wort it is all natural and you can buy it in Whole Foods or Vitamin World." Your best friend says, "Get over yourself, chill, and have a glass a wine!"

Which one is the medication?

Question 2: You are having nausea and you go to the medicine cabinet and take…. Ginger tea bought at a health food store, or anti-nausea liquid bought over the counter at the drug store, or marijuana bought on the street corner.

Which one is the medication?

Question 3: Your two year old breaks out in a diaper rash. You have a couple of choices to try. The lotion you bought at a cosmetics company. The vitamin your personal trainer said worked for her daughter's diaper rash, the oatmeal soak recommended by your doctor.

Which one is the medication?

This was a trick. They are all medications. The best definition of a medication is "ANYTHING you put in or on your body to treat a symptom, change the way you feel, or use to improve your health, no matter where you get it from."

Holistic and over the counter options are still medications. They have side effects and problems with them just like prescribed medications do. You need to watch for side effects and for drug interactions. EVERY medication that you take should be listed at your pharmacy and with your doctor in order for it to be computer checked against your prescription medications and other treatments to make sure they are compatible.

Here are the side effects of the holistic treatments listed above…
Ginger—too much can cause diarrhea, mouth irritation, heartburn, bloating, flatulence, stomach upset and sedation as possible side effects.
St John's Wort—overdose can cause fever, difficulty walking, hallucinations, and a rapid heart rate.
Oatmeal baths—those with Celiac's disease can react to the oatmeal: Bathing for more than 10-20 minutes at a time can make rashes worse.

Brown Bag Medication Review

One of the best ways to ensure that none of the treatments and medications you are using interacting with each other is to use a brown bag medication review. This is simply taking everything one has in the house used as a medication, put it in a bag, and bring it to your doctor or pharmacist to have them enter the items into your medical history. This includes ointments, dentist recommended toothpaste or mouth wash, dandruff shampoo, lotions one uses for dry skin (as opposed to a lotion that is used because one likes the smell of it). The first time people take their medications for review, 86% of them have a problem with the medications. It could be a drug interaction between the meds, it could be expired meds. If the computer shows problems, please consult the pharmacist immediately for suggestions of other options one can try. Doctors are specialists in diseases. Pharmacists have PhD levels of training on medications and chemicals. The pharmacist is always the right specialist to see when one is having trouble with or questions about any kind of medication.

Automatic Refills

So once you are sure that you are using the right medications, you need to ensure that you are taking them the right way. Sign up for the automatic refills. If one gets a phone call from the pharmacy that the medication is ready for pick up and there isn't 3 to 5 days' worth of medication left, one probably has not taken their medications every time they are supposed to. Seniors not being able to handle their own medication is the number one reason they end up in an assisted living facility. If one's goal is to stay at home as long as possible, bringing in an aide for a couple of hours a day or a week to make sure one is taking their pills correctly may be well worth the out of pocket costs.

Daily Pill Boxes

Other things you can try are the daily pill boxes. Someone comes in a puts the medications in the pill boxes by day and time of day. The senior then just needs to open the Monday morning pill box on Monday morning and take their pills. However, they do need to be alert enough to know that today is Monday. When a family choses this method to manage medications, they need to check to see if the senior is spilling meds on the floor or hiding the pills instead of taking them.

You can also try some of the new advanced systems. There are now covers you can place on pill bottles that will buzz when it's time to take that medication. There are also bigger pill dispensers that are attached to an alarm. The alarm will go off when the patient needs to take their pills. Life Alert, (the "I've fallen and I can't get up" company) and others like it, have programs where they can call into the senior's beeper and ask if they took their pills for today.

Medication management is key to a long life. So many illnesses that used to be terminal, especially related to heart problems, liver and kidney diseases, can now be managed well with medication. As I mentioned earlier, the inability to manage medications is the number one reason seniors end up in assisted living facilities. So let's figure out how to manage your medications safely and effectively and stay on top of the constant changes that aging can produce.

Chapter 9: Driver's Safety

No other topic causes so much stress for both the senior and their family than how long can they drive safely. Driving is THE thing that made Americans feel independent and grown up as a teen and so it is THE thing that says "I am no longer independent" when a senior has to give it up.

My question for everyone reading this is how many accidents after the first one before you give up your license? Having this discussion with loved ones early helps to eliminate the "decision" later on. Everyone has read or seen horror stories of seniors driving into buildings and crowds. When was the last time one saw an elderly driver driving so slowly down the road that they become the hazard? As the senior, one must be able to recognize that one's driving skills have lapsed and it may be time to give up driving. As the adult child, if the senior parent isn't willing to discuss, you must be.

I know a pair of elderly men that were best of friends. Jay (not his real name) decided he didn't feel so safe driving and he decided to leave the driving to his friend "Fred." Fred drove for about five years until he began having minor fender benders. He would back out of his garage and rip his side view mirror off his car almost every other month. He backed out of his driveway and tapped the telephone pole across the street a couple of times. He had a couple of fender benders with other cars as well. Finally, his insurance company simply said that if there was another claim on his insurance, they would cancel his insurance permanently. At that point, Fred gave up driving. Then Jay started driving again! After 5 years of not driving because he knew it wasn't safe. This is primarily because in those five years, Jay's brain had begun to change and he could no longer judge safety issues. This brain change is well documented in seniors and for American seniors it becomes the chant "I'm independent!" The more a senior brings the discussion back to independence and doing it themselves over safety, the more that shows that they are unaware of the safety issues involved. It is then that family must step up and take more control if they can. No one wants to be the adult child of the senior that crashed his car into a crowd hurting people.   Fortunately, neither of my senior friends caused serious injuries before they both gave up driving.

There are lots of reasons why seniors have more trouble driving. Aging often brings poorer hearing, lower vision, slower reflexes, and stiffness that prevent a person from turning and looking over their shoulder. Medications can make a person groggy, less alert, or down right high. Medications that have never caused a problem before can suddenly cause trouble focusing due to a mild infection or dehydration.

Additionally, seniors may not be aware of law changes. Or the state may update the way roads merge or lanes work that pits 40 years of driving familiar roads against a new way driving pattern. In my area, traffic circles are being common place, but seniors may not understand how to use them, where to turn off them, or have the ability to judge the speed of cars on the circle and may enter too soon or sit outside the circle too long. Driving too slow, the tendency of most seniors is as dangerous as driving too fast, the teenagers' problem.

Driving Help for Seniors

The good news is there are plenty of places that help seniors drive safely. AARP, local driving schools, and insurance companies all offer specialized classes designed to help seniors work around their aging bodies. In some areas, medical rehab centers may have specialized health related classes that can make modifications to a car to help a senior drive safely.

As of today, if a medical professional prescribes a medical review of driving skills, Medicare will cover the costs of both the testing and the modifications made to the car. Extra-large rear-view mirrors, cushion pads that adjust the senior in the driving seat, pads that adjust the seatbelt plus hours of re-training seniors to be more aware of their environment all is covered by Medicare. The only down side to this system is that if the senior is deemed "too poor a driver for training and car modifications to make them a safe driver" the medical rehab centers can immediately pull their licenses. On the other hand, if a loved one is that bad a driver, one doesn't want them driving anyway.

Chapter 10: Housing Options

Aging in place is the current push in senior care. Having seniors live in their original home until they pass away is the goal, as long as they are safe. While I love the idea of aging in place, my concern is always the truth of "safety."

No one would consider leaving a child under the age of 5 to stay at home for a few hours by themselves. And child protective services would be in a family's affairs if they left even older children home alone for several days. But then, we tend to be proud of our parents living alone at 80, 85, and 90. But it probably isn't a good idea from a safety perspective.

So let's look at some of those safety issues. I already mentioned that senior's brains actually change when they are isolated. They become more afraid of the outside world and that paranoia can affect the way they function in the world. If they are home alone most of the time, this is not safe for their long-term mental or social health. If one can arrange for them to get out and see people daily, staying at home is ok. If not, you might want to consider other options.

Additionally, if one's elder cannot get out of the house unassisted, they are probably not safe. Fires and emergencies happen that could require they leave the house. But if they cannot get down the stairs well or can out the door but then cannot leave the area, they may be in harms' way. One of the things I am curious about is the percentage of seniors that had to be rescued from Hurricane Harvey because they could not leave their homes unassisted. Memory problems may make it hard for them to eat appropriately, take their medications, or remember to turn off the stove. If they smoke, the risk of setting the house on fire is real.

Options for housing

Every state is a little different in how their housing options for seniors work. New York State has some of the most complicated housing options based on the senior's ability to care for himself and the cost. A quick list of options is here and we will explore some of the choices after the list.

Housing Options
1. At their home alone
2. At their home with a relative or someone else living with them
3. At a relative's house
4. In a downsized apartment or house in the community
5. In a senior retirement community-
    a. Usually these are townhomes or apartments, although there are some communities that have small houses
    b. These are divided into 2 broad categories, lower-income HUD supported or Market rate homes

6. Family-type homes- usually 2 to 6 seniors living in a traditional looking house with staff on site to keep them safe and care for their needs
7. Assisted Living and Adult Care Facilities
    a. Comes fully staffed with activities, medication management, and meals are usually provided
    b. These are again divided into two kinds, private pay and government subsidized
8. Memory Care Centers- a specialized assistant living program for those with dementia
9. Nursing Homes and Rehabilitation Centers- used for seniors who need 24 hour care of some sort. Most often that they cannot get out of a bed or wheelchair without help

All of these choices are based on what the senior can do for themselves and how close to 24-hour- a-day care they need. The first five can be done either by the senior receiving no personal or daily medical help, or the senior receiving help through a private pay agency or a Managed Long Term Care Plan (MLTC), a federal program run through Medicare and Medicaid. The last four are mostly private pay often through Long Term Care Insurance or life savings. There are some Medicaid pay options but there are few Medicaid beds available. The financial costs of the last four options often forces many families to make arrangements that are a balance of finances and safety.

I highly recommend by the time a senior is 65, they have looked closely at a couple of these options in their area. If you live in Albany, Rensselaer, Schenectady, or Saratoga County NY, you can see a complete listing of all the housing options by going online to AlbanyGuardianSociety.org and accessing their housing directory. One can either go through the directory online, or they can mail a copy that lists all four counties. One may find that the perfect housing complex for your senior is in another county. If you are not lucky enough to live in one of these 4 counties, you can check with your county department of aging or department of health to find out if there is a resource like this in your area.

Aging In Place

If a senior chooses to live at home, an aging in place specialist can help ensure safety is a priority. They can make recommendations on remodeling, moving furniture, adding grab bars, use of the latest stay at home technology or day programs that can help ensure finances alone don't dictate poor end of life care. Be open to a continuous discussion of what can be done by the senior, what can be reasonably done by family members and what needs to be hired out. Caregiver burnout is a real thing that can put the health of the primary family member giving the care in serious jeopardy, if everyone in a family isn't open to making sure that everyone has their needs met.

Chapter 11- Emergency Preparedness

This topic could be a book unto itself (and may be someday), but in the meantime, I wanted to give you a chance to think a few of these safety factors over as well.

Boil Water Advisories

Boil water advisories are issued by a town, county, or state when the public drinking water system has been potentially compromised. This is most likely been caused by a water main break, or the flooding of the sewage system during a bad storm. It could also be caused by dumping of chemicals into a local body of water from tractor trailer, train or industrial accident.

Up until a few years ago, advisories were given to the local news stations who promoted the info heavily. Nowadays, most towns do it through automated texts, emails, and robocalls. Seniors living at home may not be signed up for these services or use their emails and text system often enough to get the warning in time. They may not have the mental health alertness to realize what they need to do to keep themselves safe or they may assume they are being scammed. My mom lived with us during the last years of her life due to her dementia. When we had boil water advisories, we had to shut off the water to the house to keep her from drinking the water. This is something that might need to be done as well for a child with autism, down syndrome, or other people who may not understand what a boil water order is or remember for several hours to several days that it is in effect.

Those who live in retirement communities may be notified by their housing programs, but at the independent living levels there is no law that says they have to notify residents nor do the housing authorities legally have to be separately notified. While most staff do their best to keep up on the notifications from the town and to share it with their residents, one does need to be aware that they may not know. In NYS the Department of Health requires senior housing that is responsible for the health of their seniors (family style homes through nursing homes) must have formal plans for getting boil order advisories and ensuring their seniors are provided with healthy, safe drinking water.

When given a boil water advisory, the water from the tap must be boiled at a full rolling boil for 1 minute. Then that water must be COOLED to room temperature before it is safe, especially if the reason for the warning is the overflow of sewage into the water treatment plant. The process can be time consuming and not easily sped up. Depending on the need of the senior, one may want to keep a couple of gallons of water in the house for an emergency.

Boiled and cooled water should be used for drinking, cooking, tooth brushing, and water for pets. Washing dishes can be done by hand with a final rinse in bleach-water rinse or through the dishwasher with the drying system on heat. Ice cubes and water going through the fridge need to be dumped and the system flushed after the boil water orders have lifted. Seniors may not have the skills to clean out their water systems after the boil water orders are lifted. For further info on all the things you need to know about this, you can check Ready.gov or your state health department.

While this is crucial info for everyone to know, a senior is at more risk than others because their immune systems are more likely to be compromised by chronic illnesses. Tiny amounts of dangerous contaminants might not make the average adult anything more than mildly uncomfortable, but could make a senior violently ill. As I mentioned at the beginning, they may not get the advisory or they may not remember it is in place for the whole time. Boil water orders often last several days until the government gets two clean sets of test results.

Power Outages

Another concern is a power outage. Will the senior living on their own be safe if he suddenly wakes in the middle of the night and there is no power? Can they get out of bed and get help without falling? Will they be warm or cool enough (depending on their climate and time of year)? Will their phone work? Seniors often are unaware that phones tied to internet lines will not work without power like the old "Ma Bell" system used to. Even if they still have the old-style phone service, if they have a plug in answering machine, the phone won't work either. Many seniors have cell phones but they may not always keep them fully charged. Dementia can sneak in and make using a cell phone suddenly a challenge.

Additionally, the senior may have medical equipment that relies on power. Power companies often keep records of which people/addresses have life-sustaining medical equipment that need power. They will make an effort to get power restored or get that consumer to a safe place with power. If the electric company in your area does track, seniors should get yourself listed if they use: C-Pap machines, oxygen concentrators, powered infusion sets, suction machines, and other medical equipment that requires power. You should also check to see if your local 911, fire department, police department, or county wide senior agency has a similar program for checking on seniors.

Food Recalls

While not truly an emergency preparedness piece, spoiled food can put a senior's health at greater risk than the average adult due to chronic illnesses. Like with the boil water advisory, it is less likely the senior will be aware of a food recall. Even food that they bring home from restaurants or left over from an earlier meal may go bad and the senior not aware of it. After the age of 65, our taste buds and sense of smell begin to diminish. The senior may be completely unaware of the funky smell or taste that warns the rest of us that food has spoiled.

Tornado, Hurricane and Other Storm Warnings

As with many of these issues, the first question to ask is how will the senior living at home know this is occurring? One of the scariest moments for me was seeing an interview with an elderly man just after he was rescued from the flooding due to Hurricane Harvey. He was completely unaware that the hurricane had come through and his town was under water. This is a record setting storm that he had no idea happened outside his door.

Secondly and even more importantly, can they keep themselves safe during a storm? Can they get to a tornado shelter or the basement with their walker? If they lie down next to the bed or sofa in an earthquake, can they get back up? Will they be able to maneuver through the house to the center away from windows during a hurricane? If the basement floods during a thunderstorm, will they know and be able to get it cleaned out? Can they dig themselves out of a blizzard that dumped a foot or more of snow where they live without falling or inducing a heart attack? If one's family made plans for these occurrences, does the senior know who to get help from? These are lots of questions that only you and your family can really answer.

Evacuation Orders

Should the government give evacuation orders, how is a senior going to get out? Will they know in time to grab anything they need? Can they get out of the house with all their medical equipment, medications, and other supplies? Do they have a pet? What will they do with the pet? Is their homeowner's insurance in place? (One of the lessons learned from Hurricane Sandy was how many seniors had stopped paying their home owner's insurance.) Where are they going to go to be safe? You cannot take a senior with moderate dementia or an autistic child to a large sheltering area, they won't be safe and their caregiver will be exhausted trying to care for them in that situation.

For seniors living in family-style homes to nursing homes, the housing providers are required to have a plan for all sorts of emergency preparedness issues. The more "independent" the senior is, the less planning a facility has to do. At least in New York. If you or your loved one lives in another state, you should check their laws and regulations.

In Conclusion

Emergency Preparedness for seniors brings more questions than answers. Brutally honest answers are a requirement for complete safety, as well as staying up on the slow changes over time that alter the answers.

Have conversations now; make plans now. The earlier a senior and their family can discuss these things, make preparations, and use technology like life alerts, and safety lights that turn on when the power fails, the easier it is to continue to plan as your loved one ages. And look at repeating these conversations on a regular basis. Yearly, at least, if there have been no medical changes. After every major and minor health change it is worth reviewing. Not only for the health and safety of the senior, but for the health of the primary caregiver as well. For the peace and social health of the family. To make sure that everyone's social, spiritual, physical, and mental health are considered in the search for a perfect solution for your elderly family member's care. The conversations may even have to happen every few months or even every few weeks if you are coming closer to the end of a senior's life.

I like how one nurse described it while interviewing a patient for a Managed Long Term Care plan. "I don't care what you can do on your very best days although I am glad that you have those. In order to serve you best, I NEED to know what your very worst days look like. Because you will have more of those days as you age. And those are the days when my services might just save your life."

And as long as I have mentioned death and dying, have you, yes I mean YOU, completed a health care proxy, a living will, a last will and testament, and if you have a serious life threatening condition a MOLST form? Each of these forms provides different kinds of medical and legal protections. Just in case. Because we never know when the end is. Preparation is a good thing and help is not a four letter word. Help=Life, and a life worth living well.

www.ingramcontent.com/pod-product-compliance
Lightning Source LLC
Chambersburg PA
CBHW050801240726
48654CB00008B/578